# THE GUYS GUIDE TO THE DELIVERY ROOM

I0102024

**Edited by**

David Milne

**Published by MilHouse Publishing**
© 2011

ISBN 978-0-9559269-3-8

Nothing in this book is intended as medical advice.
It is the intention of the Author, Editor and Publisher only to
provide information of a general nature that should always be checked with a  medical profes-
sional before being acted upon in any way.

Published in 2011 by MilHouse Publishing
Balmedie, Aberdeenshire, UK

# GUY'S GUIDE
# TO THE DELIVERY
# ROOM

# Editors Foreword

When a friend of mine fell pregnant and her partner began to panic I looked around to see what information was available to help her to help him through this wonderous time that was about to happen to them. I can almost hear the women amongst you scream at me *'what* do *you mean THEM'* yes I know, it's her that is pregnant but he, the oft forgotten partner, has to undergo a lot of the events of pregnancy with her and, most importantly, is generally expected to be present at the birth these days, that is the main subject of this book.

I personally think that is a good thing, but my opinion really doesn't matter. The only problem I had with this was the almost complete lack of information for the layman, the first time father, who really has no idea what to expect during his time in the delivery room. There is a good supply of information for the women involved and so there should be, but the male of the species has almost nothing to learn from other than occasional bar room horror stories, which are not the best source of factual information.

Not being a father myself I was not best placed to do much about it personally, so I asked around amongst friends and acquaintances until I found a mother and midwife who was willing to write a guide for the completely uninitiated, the first time father. This book is her work aimed at helping the 'first time fathers to be' to understand what is going to happen once inside the delivery room.

You may find a couple of terms in here you don't understand, like 'birthing room' this is fairly new concept and is explained as necessary in the book. The other point to note is we assume that you are going to the hospital for the birth, home births are not discussed here at all and as long as you accept that there are many variations of childbirth and the basics are always the same then this book should help you understand the process a little better if not actually enjoy it.

# TABLE OF CONTENTS

# Introduction

The pending arrival of a baby is a wonderful time! It doesn't matter what the circumstances, when a new baby comes into the world, it is a true miracle. As is expected, much of the focus in the delivery room is on the woman. After all, she is the one who is enduring the pain of childbirth. What many people don't consider is that the men in the delivery room have their own issues as well.

Years ago, men weren't allowed in the delivery room. Guys were relegated to the waiting room, left to pace a hole in the floor as they waited for their offspring to be born. Today, however, there has been an enormous shift in tradition, with 90 per cent of dads now taking a hands-on approach in the birthing process.

The journey begins not only with conception but also with choosing the nursery furniture, picking out names, and taking ante - natal classes. Even with the best of training, guys may still feel out of place when attending the birth of a child. With the advent of birthing rooms taking the place of the sterile operating room, grandparents, uncles, friends, and even siblings are invited into the birth experience.

Obviously you cannot know exactly what it feels like to carry and birth a newborn; however, you can learn as much as possible about all the stages of pregnancy, labour, delivery, and newborn bonding. Perhaps once you understand the prenatal class basics you might start having doubts about how you will be able to handle it all. Try to set those uncomfortable thoughts aside. Studies show that men are more likely to get and stay involved in the care and nurturing of their children if they are present at the births.

So what's a guy to do? If you're the father to be, you have probably heard the horror stories. You're called every name in the book. You're blamed for everything from inflation to the price of petrol to getting your partner in the situation she's in. It's normal. It's probably going to happen. But how do you deal with it? That's hard to say. But the birthing experience is still something every guy can – well, not exactly enjoy, but, at the very least, participate in.

It all begins with the onset of labour. The pains begin. She screams with each contraction. What do you do? At this point, running to the store for a late night craving is out of the question. Right now, you're expected to be the supportive one. But you're confused and aren't sure exactly what to do. It can be difficult watching someone you love in pain – and childbirth IS PAINFUL! It's like a pain you, as a man, can never know.

Research shows that when a woman has a supportive birth partner, this reduces her need for pain-killing drugs and increases her satisfaction with the birth experience. This also can reduce her stresses and worries about being a mother and make her more confident after the baby is born. Having a familiar face can be very reassuring.

There are many things you can do to help the mum to be along the way to becoming a full-fledged mother. You may be confused – especially when things start getting a little frantic – and they will! With the help of this book, you'll be much more prepared for the birthing experience.

In these pages, you'll be better prepared to help with

back labour, understanding what happens in the birthing room, easing the pain of mum, and dealing with your own feelings of helplessness. It can be a daunting and scary experience, but you CAN get through it – just like SHE can!

Read on and get the definitive "Guy's Guide to the Delivery Room!"

# Changing Roles

As we've said, not so long ago, the man's place during childbirth used to be in a smoke-filled waiting room holding a box of cigars awaiting the arrival of his child. Now the opposite is true. What brought about this change?

It seems books might have had a role to play in this transformation. In 1974, Robert Bradley wrote the book Husband-Coached Childbirth, in which he basically empowered men to take as crucial a role in the birthing process as their partner (albeit not physically, of course!). At the time, Bradley was both hailed as a champion for men's rights in the delivery room and criticized as someone who was trying to advocate controlling the woman. Despite, or perhaps because of the controversy, the book 'gave birth' to the 'Bradley method' and a series of classes, still running today, in the USA.

Putting husbands in the delivery room not only coincided with feminism but also was intimately wrapped up with the natural childbirth movement and its effort to see the modern body in a more holistic fashion.

The change also could have been brought about with cultural developments. Back in the 50's and 60's, it was an unspoken rule that men just didn't go into the delivery room. However, in the 70's and 80's, men began questioning the medical status quo and took a more hands-on approach to child rearing and their rights to be present during their child's birth.

The dissolution of the nuclear family also contributed to the change with fewer women around to take care of the expectant mother's needs during childbirth. This naturally led to the man taking on that responsibility.

Changing attitudes about pregnancy in general also brought more men into the delivery room. With more and more people having children without being married as well as the rise in teen pregnancy rates, the man in the delivery isn't always the baby's father.

Today, it is almost expected that the father be present for the birth of his child. It is increasingly uncommon for the man not to participate and help out in labour and delivery. Not all men embrace this, however. Some would prefer to go back to the waiting room.

Some fathers, particularly first-time dads, feel apprehensive about seeing the woman they love in pain. Top concerns amongst expectant dads are embarrassing faux pas in the delivery room - fainting, feeling sick and squeamish and basically not knowing how to best support their partner through a potentially long and painful process.

These doubts should be considered and respected by both you and mum-to-be. It's important to think about and discuss whether you want to be present and how you see your role during the pregnancy. It can be much more complicated than it first looks.

You may both want to be together for the birth and feel very certain that this is the right thing for you as a couple. You may be concerned about whether you can cope with being at the birth as well as the intensity of labour.

You should also consider the possibility that your partner might not want you present throughout labour and birth because she doesn't want you to see her in childbirth. She may feel that she wants to be free to focus only on herself and her needs. You might quite like the idea of being her 'coach', only to find she does not want you telling her what to do.

Talking through these issues during the pregnancy can go a long way to avoid problems once labour begins. If you, yourself are unsure, talk with other guys about their experiences in the delivery room and decide that way. Just keep in mind that everyone is different and one guy's experience may not be the same as yours. Plus, if she wants you there with her, that may be your biggest deciding factor.

If you absolutely CANNOT see yourself being present for the delivery of the baby, consider a couple of alternatives. You can arrange to have another labour partner present so that if it all gets to be too much, you can leave the room either for a short time or until after the baby is born. You can choose to be present just for the labour or conversely just for the birth. You can also come in directly after the baby is born to celebrate the new life.

On the other hand is the quite clichéd but probably true problem that witnessing the physical side of the birth might not be so great for a couple's love life. This apparently happened after Elvis 'Presley became a dad for the first time. It reportedly took him months to get into the swing of things again with wife Priscilla and, shortly afterwards, their love life was allegedly non-existent. Many men can be negatively affected by what they see during delivery making it much more difficult for them after the baby arrives.

The decision about whether or not to attend the birth of your child is a personal one that should be made well prior to the onset of labour pains. Men should discuss thoroughly their feelings with their partner and both should select the option that will best suit each other.

Do not ever forget that your sole purpose at being in the birthing room is to provide strength and support to your partner. She will suffer considerable anxiety over the delivery, especially if it is her first time. She may have taken birthing classes and she may have been told what it is going to be like by a dozen different people, but until she actually experiences delivering a baby she will be apprehensive.

What a woman needs most when she's in labour is to feel safe and secure. As unprepared as men might feel, mothers can feel the same way – especially with the first baby. Support is essential, and if you won't be able to provide that, it's probably best to have someone else in the delivery room.

Some women now choose to have more than one birth partner, especially if the father might not be present. The mother should choose the person who is going to give her the support she needs. Of course, her choice must also agree to be there. Think very long and hard before you turn her down.

There's no shame in choosing the hallway or waiting room. The biggest job will come once the baby arrives, so even if you're not there from the first moment your child breathes his or her first breath, there will be plenty of time and opportunity to provide your support.

There are many birthing options these days. Not all births take place in a hospital with a doctor. Very rarely, however, will a woman be able to deliver a baby without the help of someone. We will refer to this person throughout this book as the birth attendant – whether that is a doctor, a nurse, a midwife, or a doula.

Much of the hesitation men have about being in the delivery room has more to do with lack of preparation about what to expect and training as to what they can do to help.

Let's begin by looking at the stages of labour.

# Stages Of Labour

Labour pains can come when least expected. Having a "due date" does not necessarily mean that the baby will choose that day to come into the world. The onset of labour can bring with it emotions that your partner did not expect, such as nervousness, anxiety or fear. In fact, it is at this time that a mother may not even understand what she is feeling.

Nature has designed birth simply and elegantly. Although every labour and birth is unique, and your labour will unfold in a very special way, the process is remarkably and beautifully constant.

You have, no doubt, heard the line "my waters broke". This signals the onset of true labour as the sack filled with amniotic fluid that held the baby ruptures. This can be preceded by contractions or beginnings of the contractions. Just because a woman is having contractions doesn't necessarily indicate labour, but when the water breaks, the show has started – so to speak!

Many men might wonder what contractions feel like. While we probably cannot unequivocally convey this in words, we would think that being kicked in the groin repeatedly for hours while your hair is being pulled, and your kidneys are being punched might come close. It's a pain that's hard to describe, but rest assured, it's very intense.

During the first stage of labour, the cervix softens, thins, and opens as the baby settles into the pelvis preparing for birth. The process often starts out slowly with short, infrequent contractions of the uterus. Over a period of hours or even days, the contractions become stronger and come closer together.

As the intensity of the contractions increases, the cervix dilates (becomes larger) and effaces (becomes thinner) and the baby moves lower into the pelvis. The contractions are most intense as the cervix dilates the last few centimetres. At the end of the first stage of labour, the cervix is fully opened and the baby is ready to move through the birth canal. The baby can be delivered after a woman's cervix dilates to 10cm.

The first and longest stage of labour has three distinct phases: the *early*, or latent, phase; the *active* phase; and the *transition.*

During the early phase of labour, contractions are often widely spaced—perhaps 10 minutes or more apart—and feel like a tightening or pulling in your back or groin. They can vary considerably in frequency and intensity. At this point the mother-to-be may feel excited, sociable and talkative or a bit nervous. Most women remain at home during this phase, during which the cervix dilates from 0 to 4 centimetres, and later arrive at the birth centre in active labour.

In the active phase, contractions are about 3 minutes apart lasting 45 to 60 seconds and become more centred in the abdomen. They also become stronger and more rhythmic, peaking and receding like waves. The woman's determination, at this point, may begin to wane as the reality of the impending birth presents itself. Many women think they won't be able to continue the delivery as the pain becomes stronger and stronger. This is where the birth coach becomes most important, but we'll get to that later!

Transition is the time when the cervix dilates the final two centimetres. This is the most difficult phase of labour, and produces the hardest, longest, and most frequent contractions. Fortunately, transition is relatively short, sometimes lasting for only two or three contractions. Even in a first labour, transition rarely takes longer than one hour.

During transition, contractions occur every two to three

minutes and last 60 to 90 seconds. There is little relief between them, and their intensity may cause your partner to feel frightened and overwhelmed. While she may have enjoyed your presence and physical touch throughout the early part of labour, transition may suddenly make her feel withdrawn, irritable, and short-tempered. She may develop chills, become nauseous, or feel the urge to have a bowel movement. These physical sensations reflect the descent of the baby into the birth canal and can become more intense as she enters the second stage of labour.

With a vaginal delivery, the second stage of labour is the actual delivery. When the widest part of the baby's head has settled into the birth canal, it is said to be engaged, or positioned for the delivery. At this point, contractions may slow to four or five minutes apart and become less intense. This is when pushing begins.

The birth attendant will monitor the baby's "descent" on a regular basis. When the baby's head is even with the lower bones of the pelvis, its position will be recorded as "0" station. As the baby's head continues to move through the birth canal, the stations will be identified as +1, +2, +3, etc., in reference to the baby's progress in centimetres.

Throughout the second stage of labour—which can last from 15 minutes to more than 2 hours—your baby will continue to descend through the birth canal. As the force of the contractions are combined with pushing, the baby is propelled through the birth canal. At this point, she may become very tired—especially if labour has been long or rigorous. Most women find, however, that the second stage of labour is physically and emotionally satisfying. The contractions are often easier to tolerate, and the excitement over the baby's imminent birth usually outweighs the fatigue.

As the second stage of labour progresses, the perineal

area between the vagina and rectum will begin to stretch. The birth attendant may make a small incision or episiotomy, in this region, to prevent the perineal skin from tearing during childbirth and provide more room for the baby to be delivered. We'll explore episiotomies in another chapter

As the baby approaches the bones and soft tissue of the pelvis, its pliable head will mould slightly to the contours of the birth canal. Once its head slips under the pubic bone, delivery is imminent.

As the baby's head appears, or "crowns," your birth attendant will apply subtle pressure with one hand while reaching beneath the mothers' pelvis to prepare for the baby's birth. In rare cases, forceps or vacuum extraction may be necessary to help guide the baby's head through the birth canal.

At this point, it's better for the mother to pant, rather than continuing to push, so the baby's head can be delivered gently rather than bursting out. When the head is through, your birth attendant will check to ensure that the umbilical cord remains free of the baby's neck. He or she will then immediately clear the baby's mouth and nostrils of mucus. With the next contraction, the attendant will deliver the baby's body, then clamp and cut the cord. As soon as the infant's general condition has been assessed, you will be able to cuddle and enjoy your baby.

The third and final stage of birth involves delivery of the placenta. Within a few minutes of birth, rapidly diminishing uterine contractions will cause the placenta to separate from the uterine wall. Generally, the placenta is expelled rapidly.

The birth attendant will examine the placenta, and inspect the cervix and vagina for any tears or bruises. If you have had an episiotomy, the doctor will stitch it closed. In the meantime, you and your partner will probably be oblivious to these final details as you share the joy of your new child.

So there's the beauty of birth in layman's terms. Labour and delivery can go quite quickly, or it can last for hours and hours. That's why having someone there for support is so important for the mother. It can all be very confusing and stressful. The delivery room can be a daunting place, and the procedures mind-boggling. So what happens when you first get there?

14

# Once At The Hospital

Labour and delivery can seem like a "hurry up and wait" kind of game, and most often, it is. There are things that will be done when you first arrive at the birthing facility.

Most new parents have pre-registered for their stay. If labour starts unexpectedly, you may not have had time, so, as the labour partner, you will probably have to register mum-to-be. If you're already registered, just check in (gee, just like a hotel!)

They'll then take you to your room, which these days is usually the same room where you will be during your entire stay at the hospital. That's why they are called birthing rooms. The advent of birthing rooms makes it much easier on the new parents as they aren't shuttled from here to there.

Once mum is settled into her bed, the nurse or birth attendant will check her vital signs and record them. The baby's foetal heart tones and foetal heart rate will be checked and closely monitored as these are the best indicators of the baby's response to stress during childbirth.

This is most often done by strapping an ultrasound transducer over the abdomen that will pick up the sound of the baby's heartbeat. The heartbeat will be recorded continuously on a paper strip. There will be another device strapped on top of the abdomen, which is a pressure gauge that measures the frequency and power of contractions. The combination of these two measurements will provide detailed information as to how your baby is doing during labour.

If the water has broken, the baby's condition may be monitored internally with a small electrode that is attached to the baby's head. Don't worry, this is painless and safe. This method is performed by inserting a small, spiral-shaped electrode (Foetal scalp electrode or FSE) into the vagina and attaching it to the baby's scalp to record the foetal heart rate. Usually a small catheter is placed in the uterus to measure the strength of contractions (Intrauterine pressure catheter or IUPC). This type of monitoring may give a more precise reading of the baby's heart rate and mums contractions compared to external monitoring.

Most women will also be given an IV. This is mostly done as a preventative measure in the event that medications must be administered.

The birth attendant will also do an internal examination to determine how far along the cervix has dilated. This is done very simply by inserting a lubricated, rubber gloved hand into the vagina. Early on, this is done very discreetly usually below a sheet or blanket. Resist the urge to joke at this point – no matter how strong the urge. Above all, don't tell her to "Open up and say AAHH".

The birth attendant will probably also explain what is happening and what to expect throughout the labour process. They should ask if you have questions and answer them for your peace of mind. The attendant will take some general medical information. You should be very honest about any previous medical conditions as well as any other pregnancies you have had.

Unless there's concern about complications or the risk of infection, the vaginal examination is done to check the baby's position, the dimensions of the pelvis, and the effacement and dilation of your cervix. A blood sample may be taken and a urine specimen may be tested for protein.

You should challenge any hospital procedures that seem medically unnecessary, such as extensive shaving of the pubic area or administration of an enema. There is rarely any need for these outdated rituals, but though they have been eliminated in many birth centres, they persist in some institutions.

After all this is done, all that's left to do is sit back and wait! Most birthing rooms come equipped with modern conveniences like a television set. May we advise at this point to not become more focused on a television program as opposed to the woman in pain: Many women don't look upon this behaviour too kindly.

This author has given birth twice. My first labour was filled with the sounds of the St. Louis Cardinals in the play-offs. The doctor entered the room and his first question was, "What's the score?" to which I replied through clenched teeth "7 centimetres, now turn that damn thing off!" The second was spent watching guy shows like Magnum P.I. and The A-Team. Believe me, the last thing you want to be seeing while in labour is Tom Selleck!

So what <u>can</u> you do?

# Your Role In The Delivery Room

There are many, many things you can do to help with labour and delivery. We'll address comfort measures you can offer in the next chapter. Let's first examine what makes the great birthing partner.

First and foremost, it's the ultimate show of support to attend childbirth classes prior to the delivery. This can give you a much better idea of how you can help your partner with the various stages of labour. During these classes, you will probably be given a tour of the birthing room and hospital so you can familiarize yourself with the surroundings.

Reading this book is a good starting point. Explore the process of giving birth further by finding a video and watching it and talking with others about their experiences in the delivery room.

Have the car fuelled up at all times and mechanically ready for the ride to the hospital. When labour begins, Mum may not be concentrating on much of anything other than the impending birth. Keep track of her suitcase and make sure it gets in the car with you. Be sure to call the doctor and then call relatives to let them know the baby is on its way.

Prepare yourself to be screamed at, possibly hit, and being called names you might not have ever heard of! Happily accept your punishment and don't take it personally. She's just trying to displace her pain. Remember, too, that there will be highs, lows, mood swings, and changes in behaviour that can occur at lightning fast speed. Try to keep up.

Give her lots and lots of encouragement. Tell her how wonderfully she's doing during the process. You can't say this too much. Often women will feel there's no way they can make it through the birth. It's at this point when you need to be especially encouraging and supportive. Find out what your partner's expectations are of your role in the delivery room.

Discuss your feelings and apprehensions with your partner, but be particularly sensitive to the way you do this. Instead of being sympathetic, your partner may interpret your apprehensions as a sign that you do not want to be in the delivery room.

Keep her informed. Don't chatter, but let her know how long the contractions are lasting and how long she's likely to have to relax before the next one. This is going to solely based on your personalities. Some people feel strongly that humour works well in the delivery room, but the mum who is enduring the pain and discomfort might not look at your sense of humour the same way that you do. Be sensitive to her needs above all.

Know what your partner wants before labour begins. She might not be able to communicate her wishes, so if you do it for her, she'll appreciate it. Perhaps not at that particular time, but certainly later on when it's all over with. Ask questions and get answers if you're unsure of what might be happening at a particular time.

If she gets tired, she will probably get very argumentative. Let this slide right down your back and don't fight back. She doesn't really mean it. When she feels out of control, this might be the only way she can regain it. She'll do this to you because you make her feel safe. Take it in your stride.

Don't forget to take time out for yourself. Being a labour partner can be very stressful. Take a walk around the hospital. Get a cup of coffee. Just get out from time to time to recharge your batteries. Please, however, don't do this during the end stages of labour. This could cause more problems than you'll be prepared to deal with. It would be good, too, to have a stand-in ready when you need to take a break. DO NOT; we repeat, DO NOT leave her alone for too long. You're there for support.

Be flexible when offering your support and comfort. Labour strategies that work for some women, may not work for your partner. A labour coach's job is to discern what works, and be prepared to drop what doesn't. Well before your baby's due date, you and your partner should take time to discuss her expectations and options; later you can take the initiative while keeping her wishes in mind.

Help her through transition and pushing. When contractions are doubling up and she's using every way you can think of to breathe through them (and she's too busy breathing to say anything), you can honestly tell her it will be over soon. When your partner feels the urge to push, stay close. Look her in the eyes, speak calmly, breathe with her and look happy.

Be prepared to make decisions. Only you and your partner know what you both want, but she may not be in the best condition to make hard decisions. Be ready to step in with some decisive action if the situation calls for it.

She's going to be in a lot of pain – and we mean a LOT. Don't condemn her and listen to what she needs. She'll most likely tell you before you have to act. When you think she can't bear it, she might be able to. Listen to her and react accordingly.

There's a lot going on in the birth room. Be aware of what you are willing to do during the process, and what you want to leave to the professionals. Though there will be lots of experienced people around you to whom you can look for help, you will be your partner's most important support.

This is one of those events when just showing up is the most important thing of all. Even if you want — or have — to leave most of the hands-on stuff to the pros, it will matter that you're there. Some expectant dads say they're worried they won't be up to the task, but skipping out on labour and delivery isn't an option these days.

Realize that labour is not only physical but very emotional as well. There may be moments she may not know what she wants. Just being there, respecting her, offering suggestions to change positions, or different techniques to manage discomfort, or simply embracing her and telling her she's doing great helps.

Childbirth is one of life's mysteries. Worrying is a part of that! It's normal and expected! Your baby's birthday will unfold in its own way and will have its own story. Take a deep breath and confront the fear. It will all come together. Trust yourself. Just be you. Above all, just be there!

There are many, many things you can do to ease the discomfort that she is feeling during labour. This can be the most important offering you can make, so read this section carefully and commit it to memory.

# Comfort Measures For Her

When labour begins, it's common for the mother to feel fearful. This fear leads to tension, and tension leads to pain! The more tense her muscles are (the uterus is a muscle too) the more discomfort she will have! Also, when fear is experienced, real or imagined, adrenaline is released into the bloodstream and circulated throughout the body, which affects muscle function, heat rate and causes an *increased* awareness of discomfort, anxiety, etc. There can be emotional as well as physical tension. **Relaxation is the key** in helping to facilitate the process of birth emotionally and physically.

Start finding out how she likes to be touched and/or massaged to relax before she goes into labour! Find those supporting words to whisper in her ears while she can tell you what she likes and doesn't like. Always be positive! Don't say, "You're not listening to me, not focusing, etc.!" Say, "You're doing a great job and I love you, I'm proud of you, admire you," and so on. Don't be afraid to touch her, and if she doesn't like what you're doing or saying, don't take it personally!

In the early stages of labour, try using distractions to pull attention away from the pain. Try playing a game, taking a walk, or watch a movie. Labour will progress as will the pain, but distraction early on can be an effective tool for her – and you as well!

As contractions become stronger and closer together, your role becomes more and more important. If you attended a birthing class now is the time to put all of those lessons into action. If you didn't go to a class, ask the nurse for tips.

At this point, your main job is to help keep your partner focused. She shouldn't give up, and she shouldn't panic. If she starts acting restless or agitated during a contraction, make eye contact with her and encourage her to take a deep breath. Hold her hand and tell her she's doing great.

But be prepared for the possibility that your encouragement may not be well received at times. One Edinburgh doctor recalls a dad whose wife screamed at him to shut up when he told her -- in mid-contraction -- that she was doing great.

Between contractions, you will be your partner's caretaker and servant at the same time. If she wants some ice chips, you'll be getting some – right away! If she wants a back rub, you'll be rolling up your sleeves and getting to work.

Have her eat something before going to the hospital or before heavy labour begins. We're not talking a full five-course dinner, but something to fill her belly slightly. It will most likely be many hours before she can eat anything solid, so she needs to have a little something in her stomach. Choose foods that are easy to digest and that are unlikely to cause nausea.

Once in the birthing room, create a comfortable, quiet environment with soft lighting and music. You may want to consider aromatherapy, but be warned that the senses are heightened during labour, so don't make the smells too overwhelming or intrusive.

Use loving words and touch along with a kiss or two, or three or more! Take her for an imaginary swim in a lake, or a walk on the beach to help her relax. Be prepared for her to change her mind if something isn't working for her. The best laid plans might need to be changed on a moment's notice no matter how prepared you are.

Pace yourself. You may be there for the next five or ten hours, or more, without a lot of time off. Don't forget to take care of yourself. Use your body, rather than your arms, to provide counter pressure. Sit down whenever you can.

These measures do not inhibit labour and in many cases, can enhance labour progress. Mobility and activities like pelvic rocking help the baby shift into the optimal position for birth. Upright postures allow gravity to help the baby open the cervix and descend into the birth canal. Strategies to relax muscles keep muscle tension from impeding the work of the uterus.

Some physical activities that can help with the pain include walking around, positioning pillows around her for comfort, and massaging. Many women experience severe back pain during labour. Often, rubbing her back will help alleviate the pain. One stellar trick we've learned is to bring a tennis ball to rub on her back during contractions. This saves pain in your hands and helps her with her back labour.

You may want to look into learning acupressure. Acupressure is much different than massaging. It is the application of pressure to certain points in order to alleviate pain with out rubbing and kneading the skin. This can be a very effective technique in pain management.

During periods of intense physical demand and stress, the body produces natural pain killers called endorphins. In a case of "no pain, no gain," endorphins are also responsible for the exhilaration and joy that can follow such periods. When you place pressure on certain areas, the body will release endorphins naturally.

Often, rocking will help ease the pain as well. To do this effectively, you may want to hold her from behind with your arms around her shoulders. Hold her close and gently rock back and forth in a rhythmic pattern. The rhythm will also help calm her.

It might sound like a cliché, but breathing through contractions will help immeasurably. Breathe with her and make sure she does this breathing in through her nose and out through her mouth. This will prevent hyperventilation.

Often, warm showers or baths can help with the labour pains. A great tool to have is to fill a sock with uncooked rice. This can be heated in the microwave to provide the warmth that may help relax her muscles. The alternative is a cool cloth or ice pack. Put this on her forehead or neck to provide comfort. As we've said, labour is hard work, so the possibility of her overheating is very real.

Another good technique is to have her find a spot somewhere in the room to focus on as she's breathing through her contractions. This can be something already in the room or something you've both prepared prior to delivery. Try putting the sonogram picture of your baby on the wall.

Breathing can go a long way to ease the pain of childbirth. During active labour, the goal is to remain as relaxed as possible so the cervix can continue to dilate, and provide baby with a generous oxygen supply in preparation for birth.

The following breathing techniques, used alone or in combination, can be effective throughout labour. Practice these techniques during your pregnancy. Mastering them prior to actual labour can allow you to vary the patterns to provide the most effective relief.

- **Deep, cleansing breaths.** Take these long, deep breaths at the beginning and end of each contraction.

- **Slow, chest breathing.** Take these slow, focused breaths 8 to 10 times per minute during the early, milder contractions of the first stage of labour.

- **Rapid chest breathing.** Using the same technique as you employed in early labour, double the speed of these more focused chest breaths as the first stage of labour continues and contractions increase in frequency and intensity.

- **Shallow chest breathing.** Use this shallow, panting technique at the peak of your most intense contractions.

Giving birth is a long, hard job. At some point during the hours of labour, you and your partner will discover something — perhaps a breathing pattern, a spot on the ceiling, a stuffed animal from home — that she can focus on during the contractions. With the Lamaze method of childbirth, your job is to help your partner find this distraction, and then bring her back to it whenever she starts to think she won't make it.

Always ask permission before starting anything new; you want to be sure the steps you're taking are helpful and soothing to her. Give her emotional support. Tell her often that she's doing a great job.

Using comfort measures like these delays the use of pain medication. Medications are more likely to cause problems with repeated doses, when different types of drugs are mixed, and with prolonged use. By using comfort measures, you may need only one dose of a narcotic instead of three, you may avoid using both a narcotic and an epidural, or you may delay having an epidural. We'll talk about epidurals a little later.

The benefit is that they can instantly be stopped if it doesn't help or in the unlikely event that it causes trouble. For example, if the baby doesn't like you to be in some particular position, you can simply find another one. Pain medications, once administered, cannot be rescinded, and you may need another drug or procedure to remedy the ill effects. These, in turn, introduce their own risks.

Comfort measures may not provide adequate pain relief. This can lead to a feeling of personal failure if the mother wanted an un-medicated birth. Still, this will rarely be the case if you respect and support the mother's desire to avoid pain medication, acknowledge her efforts to do so, and support whatever decision she makes. A lot of things can change once heavy labour begins so if she starts to scream for everything in the hospital's medicine cabinet, by all means, let her!

All of this takes some preparation, so you'll want to make a list before labour begins. This is often referred to as the labour "tool kit". What are some things you should include?

# The Labour Tool Kit

As the birthing partner, you'll be responsible for putting together what you'll need in the delivery room for comfort. Even though the mum-to-be is the centre of attention, you'll need some things for yourself as well.

Labour takes a long time, normally anywhere from 12 to 18 hours, perhaps longer. Most of the time labour takes place at night, so it is imperative, dad, for you to be comfortable. With that in mind it is recommended that you have a bag ready to go not only for her, but for you as well, when she announces it is time.

The good labour tool kit contains many items. Here are a few we would suggest:

- An extra shirt and/or change of clothes for yourself. You could be there awhile, so your comfort counts too!

- A bathing suit in case you want to join your partner in the bath or shower. Believe me, the sight of a naked man while in labour isn't the most welcome vision despite what you guys might think!

- Have some snacks for yourself handy. Like we've said, you could be there awhile and even if the fast food joint is "just down the road", she might not appreciate you jaunting out for a burger. Especially when all she can most likely have is ice chips or popsicles!

- A tennis ball is essential for back labour

- A portable CD or MP3 player to "set the mood" in the room

- Candles for soft lighting. Be sure to check with the hospital to see if this is allowed

- Things to do for both you and the mother. Cards, board games, word searches, crosswords, suduko and such can provide a much needed distraction during early stages of labour.

- If the doctor will allow it, bring lollipops for her to suck on when she gets hungry.

- A list of phone numbers for the people you'll want to call once the blessed event occurs. We have one note about calling people after the blessed event.

As a general rule men want to know two things, what the sex of the baby is and is mum doing well. The details are unimportant.

Women, however, require details. Having a baby is a defining event in a woman's life; it is also a benchmark by which women compare themselves to one another. Therefore, you have to provide certain extra information to women. Understand that what you provide is not nearly enough, but coming from a man it will be more than they expected and will be appreciated; they will also brag about you to your wife and ALL your female friends.

Scented oils and lotions can help soothe the nervous mother while you're rubbing the areas she needs massaged.

DON'T FORGET THE CAMERA! Most hospitals don't allow video cameras in the birthing room anymore, but they encourage picture taking – especially after the baby arrives. If you're bringing a digital camera, don't forget plenty of batteries!

Change for the vending machines. In case your snacks give out!

What happens if the comfort measures don't work and Mum needs some medication? Most likely, it's an epidural. Let's define some non-natural pain relief.

# Pain Medications

Making the decision to have a natural childbirth is every woman's personal decision, but often they change their mind when the reality of the pain they are experiencing hits them.

I had both of my children naturally, but I was young and naïve. If I were to have a baby today, I would choose medication. With the medical technologies out there today and the advances made in medicine, having a little extra relief just makes sense.

At any rate, there are two basic medicinal relief's that can be made during labour to ease Mum's pain. These are pain relievers (much stronger than Tylenol or Asprin) and the epidural. We'll look at both.

## Pain Relievers

All drugs cross the placenta to the baby, and therefore it makes sense to use them only when necessary, and in the smallest yet the most effective dosages. Nubain and Demerol, for example, are common medications to give in labour. They are given in small dosages but they do tend to decrease the effort of the uterus and they may make the baby sleepy if given too close to the delivery.

Intrathecal morphine is a newer system of pain relief which is gaining wider acceptance. Morphine is instilled through a catheter into the space next to, but not within, the spinal cord in the lumbar region. Foetal effects are minimal and the mother attains excellent pain relief without losing uterine effort while still maintaining the pushing reflex. Side effects include itching and nausea in some patients.

The doctor may offer to do a para-cervical block. Medication is injected into the cervix, usually during the first stage of labour, to provide pain relief from contractions and dilation without interfering with the urge or ability to push. This drug may not work properly in up to one-third of women, and it must be repeated every hour to maintain numbness. It is not used frequently today.

A Pudendal block is another option. The anaesthetic is injected through the vaginal wall during the second stage of labour to relieve pain in the perineum (the area between the vagina and the rectum). It may be used in an otherwise un-medicated childbirth. The medication does not interfere with the urge or ability to push and generally masks the effects and repair of an episiotomy—the incision made to enlarge the vaginal opening.

Finally, there is the spinal or saddle block. A single injection of regional anaesthetic is made into the spinal canal, numbing the complete lower abdominal and perineal area. This type of anaesthetic is rarely used during labour but may be suggested if a forceps or caesarean delivery is required. Administration of a spinal block completely removes the urge to push and may lower blood pressure. In rare cases, it causes a severe headache when it wears off.

## Epidurals

The epidural is gaining in popularity to ease the pain of childbirth. A needle holding a thin, flexible tube is threaded into the space between the spinal cord and vertebrae. When the needle is removed, the anaesthetic can flow continuously through the tube.

Like a spinal block, this procedure provides full pain relief in the perineal area. Dosages can easily be changed or discontinued. Most physicians consider the epidural block to be the optimal method of pain relief for uncomplicated labour or non-emergency caesarean births because it allows a woman to remain fully alert. Nevertheless, the anaesthetic requires up to 20 minutes to take full effect and may leave a painful "hot spot". In addition, it may diminish uterine contractions, bringing on the need for oxytocin. The risk of a forceps delivery is also increased.

An anaesthesiologist will be called in to administer the medication and place the tube. Generally, the only people allowed in the room during the procedure will be the mother, the birth attendant, and the doctor. You may be allowed to remain as well, but if you're not, don't worry.

The anaesthesiologist will have the mother sit up on the bed for the insertion of the tube. She may be given a numbing shot first in the spinal area. It's important that she remain completely still during the procedure to avoid any problems with the insertion of the needle and tube. It doesn't take very long to do the procedure, so this generally isn't a problem.

Epidurals are a necessary and excellent option for some women. They work best in women with prolonged labours. Most women can tolerate a labour which is progressive. But after many hours of minimal progress, when her support people are fading from exhaustion, when she is feeling as if all her work is not achieving her goal, the type of analgesia provided by the epidural allows a mother to rest and regroup.

She should be counselled to expect IVs, artificial rupture of membranes, confinement to bed, oxytocin augmentation and that the use of internal or external foetal monitoring will now be necessary. Such interventions come at the price of 'medicalising' the experience and taking away some of her control over her experience. For some this is a small price to pay for relief of pain and they feel that they do get some control back when pain is relieved.

Nearly all women who have chosen the epidural have reported being glad that they did – almost to the point of giddiness. This is especially true of women who aren't having their first child and declined the epidural the first time around. I think the phrase I've heard is along the lines of, "If I had known it would have been that great, I wouldn't have hesitated!"

OK, we've made it into the birthing room and we know how to give Mum some comfort measures along with possible medication options. What about when it comes time to push?

# Delivering The Baby

Once the woman's cervix is fully dilated to 10cm, it will be time for her to push. For many guys, this may seem like an easy task. After all, it's just pushing. Well, remember that a baby is a lot bigger than the hole it's coming out of. I once heard a comedian say it's like a man pushing a bowling ball out of his nose.

At any rate, this doesn't go as quickly as you might think. The delivery part of childbirth is the hardest part – even harder than putting up with the pain of contractions!

This is where your resiliency really comes into play. The big thing men need to remember about delivering a baby is that – well – it's gross, but beautiful all at the same time. Many guys report that they didn't mind the contractions and heavy labour, but when it came to the actual delivery, they were completely taken aback.

The most often heard advice in locker rooms when talking about being present during childbirth might be to stay at the head of the bed and don't look down. It's a matter of choice, but this is a one time thing, so if you really, really don't want to watch, don't. But be aware that you might miss out on something wonderful!

It's at this time when her legs will be splayed apart and everything God gave her will be exposed. Believe me, she doesn't care. Her modesty went out the door when the baby bore down in her pelvis trying to get out.

When she is having a contraction is when she should be

pushing. The birth attendant will be extremely helpful during this time and listening to them is very important. You will get into a rhythm, though.

The general position for pushing is with the legs apart – big surprise there, huh? She should take a big breath in through her mouth, hold it, put her chin to her chest and bear down. Pardon the description, but it's like taking a big, huge – um – bowel movement (to be as general about it as we can be!)

Every time she pushes, the baby travels a little further down the birth canal. Breathing during the push causes the baby to "suck back" just a little and impedes the progress, so encourage her to keep pushing as long as she can.

When labour really gets underway, she will be asked to do this three times in a row for 10 seconds at a time. This means the process will be something like this: deep breath, push while you count to ten (one-Mississippi, two-Mississippi, etc.), a short rest and then again two more times. The more she does this, the more progress the baby makes. If she holds her breath, this will provide more strength behind the pushing.

However, there really is no one "right" way to push or breathe. It depends on what her body is telling her. Just be by her side and support whatever adjustments she needs to make in order to make the process progress.

What do you do at this point? Hold her legs behind the knees bringing them up to her chest, count, and encourage! You can't say "You can do it" enough times. You can also try phrases like "Keep it up", "You're doing great", "That's the way to do it", etc.

Some phrases to avoid include "Wow, that's gross",

"Can't you do any better than that", "It can't be that bad", and "Get it out for heaven's sake, Sports Centre is coming on". (Sorry, I just had to inject a little humour there!)

While she's pushing and you're counting, the birth attendant will be monitoring the baby's progress again with the lubricated, gloved fingers. They will probably also be making a circular motion around the cervix to make room for the baby.

The doctor may choose to do an episiotomy to help provide a little more room for the baby come out. This isn't nearly as bad as it seems, but you should know about it.

# Episiotomies

An episiotomy is done by snipping the bottom of the vaginal opening to enlarge it for birth. With a midline or median episiotomy, the usual type in the U.S. and Canada, the practitioner cuts straight down toward the anus. With mediolateral episiotomy, the preferred type in other parts of the world, the cut slants off to one side. Some U.S. and Canadian caregivers routinely do mediolateral episiotomies, and some do them under certain circumstances such as for forceps deliveries.

According to the US medical profession, midline episiotomies are easier to repair, hurt less afterwards, cause less blood loss, cause fewer complications during healing, give better anatomical results, and are less likely to cause pain during intercourse. However, midline episiotomies are much more likely to extend into or through the anal sphincter.

If the baby is in trouble close to the birth, the doctor or midwife will not want to wait the additional time it may take for the birth without an episiotomy. In some cases a woman is exhausted or not stretching well and the caregiver will recommend an episiotomy. However, unless the birth attendant rarely does episiotomies, that judgment is questionable. If exhaustion is the issue, remember that an episiotomy shortens labour by an average of nine minutes – and that's a good thing!

Many birth attendants hesitate to do episiotomies. Some believe that they lead to pelvic floor weakness. The pelvic floor is a complex group of muscles that form a hammock suspended between the pubic bone in front and the base of the spinal column in back. The urethra, vagina, and anus all pass through it. Pelvic floor weakness or injury can lead to sexual dysfunction, urinary stress incontinence, and anal incontinence.

However, if the baby just isn't going to come out with an episiotomy, it becomes absolutely necessary, and most women heal easily from the procedure with Kegel exercises to strengthen the cut muscle.

There will be some discomfort in the first few days after childbirth even without an episiotomy. It is common for there to be some general soreness or even a small injury to the perineum. However, having an episiotomy will greatly increase the chances of having enough pain to interfere with walking or sitting comfortably. There can also experience intense stinging with urination and moving your bowels can be very uncomfortable for the first few days.

If you are unfortunate enough to have one of the complications of episiotomy -- it extends or infects -- you could be looking at a prolonged period of pain, or problems such as anal incontinence that could seriously or even permanently affect your quality of life, especially in having sexual relations.

The harm done by episiotomy may also not show up immediately. Urinary and anal incontinence may only begin years later when aging and further childbearing add to the toll taken by episiotomy.

Then the baby arrives.

# The Baby Arrives

There's really not much that can be said about the actual birth of the baby. As we've told you, there's a lot of pushing, screaming, grunting, and yelling (well, most of the time!) prior to the arrival. We'll do the best we can, though!

After all this pushing, the baby's head will begin to "crown" or show at the edge of the vagina. It's at this time that Mum will be asked to push with all her might. It's hard work bringing a baby into the world, and at this point, it gets much harder. For the guy reference, read back to the "bowling ball" comment!

The baby has made its journey down the birth canal and is close to entering the world. Once the baby's head is out, Mum is usually asked to stop pushing at which time the birth attendant will use a plastic bulb to suck out the mucus from the nose and mouth.

After the head comes the shoulders and baby is here! This all happens very, very fast, so if you want to witness the baby's birth, be sure to focus your attention there. Mum is beginning to feel a huge sense of relief even after the head presents, so she's doing alright.

The baby will be covered in mucus, so don't be alarmed. It washes off. Many men feel newborn babies resemble the traditional view of what aliens would look like. Please refrain from saying anything of this sort. Mum's just worked her butt off bringing that alien into the world, so keep it to yourself. Besides, that look wears off quite quickly and the baby turns into the most beautiful human being ever created. Trust me!

The umbilical cord will be clamped off and then cut. You may be asked if you want to cut the cord. That's your decision but rest assured it doesn't hurt baby or mum at all.

There are times when it is necessary to help the delivery

along using forceps or a vacuum extractor. Forceps resemble two large salad spoons, and the doctor uses them to guide the baby's head out of the birth canal.

Vacuum extraction is done with a soft plastic cup that looks similar to an ice cream cone, and it is applied to the baby's head and stays in place by suction. There is a handle on the cup that allows the doctor to use this to assist with delivery through the birth canal. The choice between using forceps or a vacuum extractor is usually made by the doctor. Neither of these procedures will cause baby harm, so don't be alarmed.

This is the big moment, an event you'll remember for the rest of your life. And here's the tough part: You must STAY CALM. Try to save your tears and hysteria until after the baby is born. Your wife needs your support, figuratively and literally.

You'll be giving her encouragement with every push, and you may also be supporting her back so she can push comfortably. If you're up to it, you should also take a few moments to watch the actual birth. When you get your first glimpse of your baby's head, you can reassure your partner that she's almost done.

When the baby is born, he or she will generally be placed on mum's stomach and you'll get the first really good look. There's a reason why doctors place the baby there.

When newborns are kept close to their mother's body, they apparently feel safe, and the transition from life in the womb to existence outside the uterus is made much easier for them. The newborn also recognizes his mother's voice and smell, and her body warms his -- faster and in a healthier way than if placed in a bassinet fully covered with blankets or in an incubator.

When full-term infants are skin to skin with their mother, they very seldom cry during the first 90 minutes of life. However, when placed in a nearby bassinet, they cry about 20 to 40 seconds during every five-minute period for the next 90 minutes. Newborns are already perceptive enough to know the difference between a bassinet and their mother!

Once the baby is here, ask Mum what she needs for you to do. Does she want you to start calling people or does she just want to sleep – or both?

Help her relax. She may still benefit from back rubs, and she'll still be feeling some pain. Above all, enjoy the moment! Except for feeding and loving your baby, this is a time to rest. There's plenty of time later to think about the last 18 hours and the next 18 years.

Men often have two impulses after watching their child being born. First, they cry. Then they grab a camera. As your partner holds your baby for the first time, you'll be firing the flashbulb. After a few good shots, you'll want to put down the camera and pick up your baby. Hold him close and let him study your face.

If your baby goes to a nursery while your partner recovers, go along and keep him company. When he drifts off to sleep, you can make the first round of phone calls to friends and family. And don't forget to check in with your partner, too. If she's awake, she'll want to hear the very latest on the baby's condition. She'll also want to hear how great she was.

And that's about it. For all the work and pain, there's now a beautiful new life to celebrate! What happens to baby right after birth?

# Procedures For The Baby

The period immediately after your baby's birth will be an exciting, awesome and exhilarating experience. In these moments, with your baby close to you, all your dreams, hopes and plans come together.

At one minute after birth, the paediatrician or labour nurse will assign your baby an Apgar score. This score helps the medical team assess if the baby needs oxygen or other forms of medical support. Another Apgar score will be given at 5 minutes of age.

It is very important to keep newborns warm. Your baby will be wrapped in blankets and perhaps placed in an open warming crib.

The surgical clamp used on the umbilical cord will be switched for a small plastic clamp, similar in appearance to a hair barrette, and the cord end will be trimmed. Within the first day of birth, the stump of the umbilical cord may be treated with a purple dye to prevent infection.

The birth attendant will take the baby's vital signs and check for any possible complications. The baby will be cleaned, weighed, and measured.

Some US state laws require that an antibiotic be placed in baby's eyes. This is to prevent blindness from maternal vaginal infections. Most hospitals use Erythromycin ointment, but some still use silver nitrate, which can be more irritating. This does not always happen elsewhere in the world

An injection of Vitamin K will be given in the thigh. This vitamin is needed by the liver to assist with blood clotting. In the adult, bacteria in the intestines manufacture vitamin K. Newborns have no bacteria in their intestines; consequently, they are not able to produce vitamin K on their own. Vitamin K injection prevents bleeding problems in the newborn.

A blood sugar test might be necessary if the baby is very large or very small or if Mom had gestational diabetes. Usually, the nurse or phlebotomist pricks the baby's heel to get a drop of blood. If the baby's blood sugar (glucose) is too low, Mum may be asked to nurse baby or give him/her some formula or sugar water.

You can make some huge brownie points after baby arrives by pampering Mum at this point. Mum has been through a lot both physically and emotionally. Now is a good time to show her how much you love her. Bring flowers, splurge on chocolates, or write her a love note. Whatever you do, find a special way to mark the occasion.

However even the best laid birth plans can go awry and a caesarean birth becomes **necessary**.

# Reasons For A Caesarean Birth

The rate of caesarean births in the United States has sky-rocketed from 5 percent in the 1960s to nearly 25 percent since the 1980s. Many factors have contributed to this increase, including the frequency of repeat caesarean delivery, the use of electronic foetal monitoring, the declining use of vaginal breech and forceps deliveries, and the drift toward surgical intervention for "failure to progress" in labour.

While caesarean delivery is certainly safer today than during the 1960s and obviously indicated in extremely high-risk situations or emergencies, it still causes a higher rate of maternal injuries than vaginal delivery.

Caesarean delivery is often accepted as the inevitable outcome to a complication arising during labour. Based on the experience of the past two decades, however, most experts agree that surgical intervention is not always in the best interests of the woman or baby. In order to make an informed decision, it's important to understand some of the common complications that can occur during labour.

## Premature Rupture

Most women begin labour spontaneously when their membranes rupture and their pregnancies have reached full term. When labour does not begin within 12 to 24 hours, the situation is described as "premature rupture of the membranes" (PROM). Because PROM certainly plays a role in high caesarean rates, more doctors are proceeding with a quick induction of labour after a PROM at full-term.

Although the "wait-and-see" approach has been associated with fewer caesarean deliveries than the use of oxytocin to stimulate contractions, one large study has concluded that induction of labour using vaginal suppositories containing prostaglandin E2 is a viable option for handling PROM—especially in women experiencing a first labour. In the study, the rate of caesarean section in the women who received prostaglandin was half that of those who either received oxytocin or waited for the onset of labour.

## **Failure to Progress**

Physicians generally agree that once active labour has begun, a woman's cervix should dilate 1.2 cm to 1.5 cm per hour. Sometimes dilation falters during the active phase despite regular contractions. This condition is known as "failure to progress."

Because labour can be interrupted for a variety of reasons, the immediate cause is not always clear to the woman or her physician. Should this occur, the doctor will perform a pelvic exam, check vital signs, and monitor the baby for a short period of time. If all appears well he or she can take a hands-off approach or consider the possibility of "actively managing" your labour.

A number of procedures are effective in re-establishing labour. If the amniotic sac has not yet broken, the doctor may suggest breaking it manually, a procedure known as amniotomy. Because rupturing the membranes commits a woman to delivery, this can be a risky strategy during the latent phase, when false labour is always a possibility.

Several research studies have concluded, however, that amniotomy performed during active labour actually shortens its duration by up to 2 hours. Moreover, the rate of vaginal delivery increases, and there is no added risk of injury to the woman or baby.

Doctors disagree on how to handle the 10 percent of

pregnancies that extend beyond 40 weeks. The main goal is to avoid injury or death to the baby due to lack of oxygen or intake of meconium in the lungs—established risks in post-term pregnancies. Some doctors advocate inducing labour at 41 to 42 weeks, while others recommend foetal monitoring until labour begins spontaneously.

In one large study of women with post-term but otherwise uncomplicated pregnancies, the induction of labour resulted in a lower rate of caesarean delivery, mainly because there was less foetal distress. In any event, few clinicians allow a pregnancy to continue past 42 weeks. In these rare instances, labour is often induced with prostaglandin gel or oxytocin.

## Pelvic Size

Certain variations in a woman's anatomy also can lead to complications during labour. During vaginal delivery, the baby must be propelled through the pelvic area by the contractions of the uterus and "bearing down."

In general, a woman's pelvis is large enough and shaped properly to allow for the baby's passage. In fact, unless she has a history of pelvic fracture or bone or neuromuscular disease, the physician should not discourage her from trying a natural delivery strictly on the basis of pelvic dimensions. Even if her pelvic area is smaller than average, it may still be big enough for the baby if the rest of labour progresses normally.

Nevertheless, in some cases, the size of the baby's head does exceed the dimensions of the birth canal. If this happens, labour will almost certainly fail to progress during the second stage; and the first stage of labour may be irregular as well. If the size of the baby is the cause of a woman's "failure to progress," she will need a caesarean.

# Position of the Baby

In more than 95 percent of full-term labours, the baby's head is "presenting" —pointed toward— the cervix. Typically, the baby's head is tucked against its chest, with the crown of the head facing the birth canal in preparation for delivery.

In some unusual situations, a baby's face, forehead, or top of the head is presenting. If the baby remains in either of the latter two positions throughout labour, a caesarean delivery may be necessary since the broadest part of the baby's head may be too wide to clear your pelvis.

A full-face presentation is very rare. Unless she's already had several children, the physician will almost certainly insist on caesarean delivery should this occur. Vaginal delivery increases the risk of injury to the baby's neck or spinal cord.

The position—or attitude—of the baby is another consideration in determining the safest method of birth. More than 99 percent of the time, a full-term baby lies vertically in the uterus. In the remaining cases, known as a transverse lie, the baby's back faces the birth canal. A baby in this position when labour begins almost always must be delivered by caesarean.

Caesarean sections are surgery, so special procedures must be taken as opposed to a vaginal delivery. You can still be present for the birth, but you should know what to expect.

# Guys Guide To A C-Section

Preparation for the surgery includes starting an IV, shaving the pubic hair that shows when your legs are together and inserting a bladder catheter. Her belly will be washed with antiseptic and sterile drapes placed around the incision site. A blood pressure cuff and sensors will be put on her chest and finger to monitor blood pressure, heart rate and blood oxygenation. A curtain will be hung across her upper chest so that she cannot see the operation.

Most caesareans are performed under epidural anaesthesia because it is safer than general anaesthesia. If an epidural is already in place, the anaesthesiologist will strengthen it so that she is numb from the toes to the breastbone.

You will first be asked to change into surgical scrubs. Upon entering the operating room, you will be given a place to sit near the head of the operative table. You will probably also be told not to touch anything that is a part of the "sterile field" for surgery- this is very important, like an airline pilot asking you not to touch the controls once the plane is in the air! The two of you will be able to talk as the operation progresses, which will be reassuring to you both.

If you wish, you can look over the drapes and observe part or all of the caesarean; her doctor will direct you. It's particularly special to see the baby emerge from the uterus, which is not as yucky as it sounds. Both of you should be able to hear your baby's first cry shortly after it's born; if you didn't find out the baby's sex before birth, your doctor will announce the answer at this time. The baby is then handed to the paediatric staff to be dried off, evaluated, and given medications; these duties are essentially the same as with a vaginal birth.

If general anaesthesia is used, she will be put under by

injection of a medication into her IV. Once unconscious, the anaesthesiologist will put a tube down her throat to maintain an airway and deliver a gas aesthetic

The operation generally takes an hour or so. The time from beginning the operation until birth of the baby is typically about five minutes. The greatest part of the time spent after the delivery is for suturing the various tissue layers.

With rare exceptions, the roughly four-inch incision is made horizontally just above the pubic bone. A horizontal uterine incision is preferred because it produces a much stronger scar. However, in certain situations, such as when the placenta is covering the cervix, the incision is made vertically.

During the surgery, she will feel pulling and tugging but no pain. The manipulations could make her queasy, so reassure her that this is normal.

After the delivery, the obstetrician hands off the baby to be examined. Some hospitals permit healthy babies to remain with your partner and you during the rest of the operation. In others, staff will take the baby to the nursery, regardless of the baby's condition.

As the hospital staff examines the newborn, the obstetrician delivers the placenta through the incision, suctions out fluid and begins closing the uterus and inner tissue layers with stitches. The skin incision may be closed with conventional stitches, staples, or even with tape strips. Finally, the surgical wound is covered with a dressing

After the surgery, she will be taken to a recovery area where she can be closely monitored for the next couple of hours. In some hospitals, the staff will bring her the baby to hold and breastfeed. Policies vary as well as to whether your can be with her in recovery and whether may be in the nursery with the baby.

The next day, she will continue the dual duties of healing from major surgery and beginning to care for your new child. This recovery process begins with starting to walk again, dealing with pain from the surgery, and awaiting return of her "bowel function" (so she can eat). Your encouragement and assistance will be needed frequently at this time.

A post-operative stay in the hospital requires an average of three days, but your partner will still be feeling the effects of the operation long after she goes home- usually another five to seven weeks. Your willingness to help out, understanding that she is exhausted and uncomfortable, is vital to the beginning of your new family.

If Mum has had to have an unplanned caesarean- in other words, one decided upon because labour hasn't progress normally- she will also have to deal with her feelings caused by not having a "natural birth."

Many women interpret this as a FAILURE, even if they couldn't have done anything to prevent it (which is almost always the case). Be aware of this emotional reaction, and encourage her to talk about it. The most helpful reaction to her comments is often just listening without interrupting. If her negative feelings persist for more than a few days, make sure her doctor knows.

That's some pretty graphic stuff we've given you above. So what are the downsides of being in the delivery room?

# Deciding To Be There Or Not

Even though most men are expected to be present for the birth of their child, many are more than reluctant to do so. We feel it's important to consider the downsides to being present for the birth of the baby.

As we said earlier, probably the number one reason men don't want to be around for birth is they tend to view their partners in different ways once a baby has come from the "pleasure area".

One quote we've seen seems quite appropriate.

*"If an area that's zoned for recreation gets rezoned for business, it's hard to get it zoned back".*

There's a huge psychological shift that occurs after a man has seen his partner give birth. In bed, she suddenly becomes someone's mother instead of the sexual being he was once with.

This is usually not a long-term problem however. Men are sexual beings and when she wants to have sex, they can usually "kick it into overdrive" and succumb to his own natural instincts. When you're not having sex, you've got all that time to think about why you're not, so you can come up with a thousand reasons. But rest assured if she is ready to have sex, all those issues go right out the window.

Witnessing childbirth tends to take some of the mystery out of sex and her "private" parts. Breastfeeding can complicate this even further.

When a woman is lactating, her breasts can become weapons much like the Fem-Bots in the Austin Powers movie. Breast milk is replenished with stimulation. If this is part of your foreplay, be prepared to be "squirted" from time to time - as gross as that might sound.

While this might sound hopeless, it really isn't. These feelings can be overcome. You don't have to endure intense therapy to regain your sex life after child birth.

Generally, doctors recommend abstaining for six weeks after the birth of the child. There are some steps you can take to re-claiming the pleasure of your sex life.

First, remember that you helped make that baby. Nature made her the one able to give birth. Her body was constructed for that purpose, but it was also constructed to bear children, so look at it as a natural course of events.

Her body will regain its allure in time and you will be attracted to her again. That's how we can explain couples with more than one child! As the sensitive, caring man that you are, there are steps you can take.

Reinforce her efforts as a mother- especially if it's her first time. Nature requires her to place her first priority on getting her offspring off to a good start, and she won't relax until she feels successful with that. If she seems chronically worried or depressed about how she's doing as a mother, let her doctor know.

Share in the baby-care duties as much as she wants you to, even at night. Remember that she's got a new baby, and is healing from a major surgery, so she will be exhausted and uncomfortable- and that's not very romantic. Plus, this will show you are a caring partner who wants to actively take part in the job of parenting.

Encourage her to exercise: reinforce any efforts she makes, and help her free up time to exercise. As she starts feeling good about her body, her sex drive will naturally increase. (Note that she will need to follow her doctor's advice about exercise, which will restrict her for at least six weeks.)

Don't forget romance! It's easy to fall into a pattern of tag-team baby care technicians, and forget the mutual attraction that got you to make a baby in the first place. Although patience is required, when the time is right, a nice dinner out or a weekend away for the two of you should help re-ignite that old flame.

Remember why you were attracted to her in the first place. We're willing to bet it had little to do with her "business parts". Focus on that and keep the memory of child birth out of the bedroom.

Once you become parents, it becomes very difficult for both partners, to find time to spend together as a couple. A newborn baby takes up all the time of both the mother and the father. Though it may seem that the baby is affecting your relationship, it is not so. A baby doesn't damage a good relationship and a baby doesn't improve a bad one. It is ultimately up to the partners to find time for each other no matter how difficult it is or how tired they are.

For some time each day continue to think of your partner as your lover and not the father or mother of your child. Spend time with the baby together, play and cuddle the baby together. This will give you quality time together and as a family. Once a week ask a friend or a family member to take care of the baby for a few hours so that both of you have time together alone.

Your sexual relationship maybe affected to a great extent once the baby is born. Since this important aspect of your relationship is affected this may take a toll on your relationship. As a new mother the demands of the baby, exhaustion, unhappiness with bodily changes after childbirth and the effect of breastfeeding on sex drive all affect her sex drive after birth. Your partner may feel that you have only time for the baby and not for her. While you may feel that everyone is only making demands on you and you don't have any time to rest or to yourself. Making time to improve your sexual relationship will help you and your partner.

Just remember, there is no right time to restart your sex life. Intercourse is not always necessary. Just lying together, cuddling together and spending time together can improve your relationship and make you comfortable with your body. If sex in painful even after healing then don't do it. Consult your doctor and let them advise you what to do.

Above all, remember that the vagina is an elastic and supple tissue, which heals quickly and a woman's body was created to bear children. The human body has great recuperation powers. Unfortunately, the human mind tends to dwell on other issues. Work on looking at your partner in a different way when it comes to romance and love making.

# Conclusion

As we have said before, the decision whether or not to be present for the birth of your baby is a very personal one that must be made individually. We do not want to sway you one way or another.

There is a continuing debate on whether or not men should be allowed in the delivery room. Some feel that they cause more problems than they solve. It has even been said that over-anxious expectant fathers are the cause for the increase in c-sections because they cannot stand to see their partner in such pain.

On the other side of the coin, many men feel like they are useless in the delivery room. They really have little concept in understanding what the woman is going through, and simply stand by until someone tells them what to do.

The miracle of watching a new life enter the world, while wonderful, can be equally startling and even disturbing for some men. While most dads are able to eventually forget the more graphic images, not every man gets over it.

Even though you're in the delivery room, that doesn't mean you necessarily have to have the same vantage point as the doctors and nurses if that what you're worried about. You can still be in the battle without being on the front lines!

It is miraculous to see a baby's head emerge, and it can also be shocking. It is riveting to see an umbilical cord connecting mother and baby, but it can also be very disturbing. It is exciting to be asked by a doctor to cut that umbilical cord, but also potentially very frightening, even for otherwise rather fearless men.

It is rare to hear a father say that he wished he had not been present for the birth of their child. The only time a father in the delivery room could present a problem is when he could simply not bear to see his wife in pain and because of this brought to the birth a sense that the discomfort his wife was experiencing was not normal and was somehow his fault.

No one likes to stand by helplessly while someone they love is in pain. This is why preparation classes are so important. The partner plays a definite role in assisting the birthing woman and enables her to cope more effectively.

But if you don't feel you can handle watching your partner in extreme pain, don't do it. If you get squeamish just by the thought of witnessing childbirth, stay in the waiting room. The big part of this is to discuss it wholeheartedly with your partner.

You may be pleasantly surprised at her reaction. She may be relieved and invite in her mother or her best friend with the knowledge that they can, in fact, handle the drastic and often disturbing images that accompany bringing life into the world.

Labour and childbirth is not something that happens *to* a woman, but *what* a woman *does* all by herself. There is no outside "force" that descends upon her to *make* her experience childbirth and the discomforts associated with it! It is a natural, innate, physiological process!

A woman's body is magnificently designed, physically and *chemically* to birth a baby. The discomfort comes from various physiological processes including pressure on anatomical structures, tissues stretching and from natural contractions that are much kinder than those stimulated by pitocin. And the hormones in her body make it happen!

Your job is to help her through the process in any way you can. Be her guardian. Protect her privacy, her wishes. Ask questions and do what SHE needs for you to do.

If you've never been in a delivery room before, you may feel uncertain about your job. Are you supposed to be a cheerleader, a coach, or an unofficial nurse? It's usually a little bit of everything. Your partner will need you at every stage, from the first contractions to the delivery and beyond.

While this book is a great start, you can get some great hands on experience by enrolling in a child birth class. They are usually offered through your local hospital and almost always have convenient times to accommodate most schedules.

As we've outlined many techniques, you will learn ways to relax her and massage her, what positions to use, and when to use warmth and cold on her body to reduce discomfort and so much more! AND PRACTICE, PRACTICE, PRACTICE the skills you learn!

These classes are invaluable because education is proactive! When you learn about something new, it gives you the information and the confidence you need to do what you have learned. When you are an active participant, it gives you a sense of control as well as personal satisfaction. Imagine how great you'll feel knowing you knew how to help her because you had the knowledge. (Also, the relaxation techniques you learn, you can do them too! It will help you to relax as well and throughout your life.)

Your role is very important. Your physical presence and emotional strength mean a lot to your partner's feelings of security. And what you do to support your partner through labour and birth will reassure her that you're going to be with her every step of the way.

Don't let fear hold you back from being there for your

partner – and your child! Be proactive about this incredible event! Learn all you can about it! As *you* learn more, you will be more comfortable with your role in, during and with your partner's experience during labour. In the end, you'll both share a fantastic achievement -- the birth of your baby! There are A LOT of things you can do!

When it comes down to it, you will only get one chance to welcome the new life you helped to conceive into the world, and that moment is the seconds after birth. The place is in the delivery room. As soon as you can hear, touch, and smell your newborn, you enter into a whole new world—the world of fatherhood. It will be full of challenges, but it will also be full of the most precious gifts in life!

The following websites were referenced in researching this book:

www.healthsquare.com
www.drspock.com
www.babyworld.com
www.dadstoday.com

# Notes

# Notes

# Notes

# Notes

# Notes

This book is a product of MilHouse Publishing who can be contacted via their website at www.milhousepublishing.com, which is also where you can see some of the other products they have available.

Some of these are shown on the next few pages:-

"Blinded by the Bling??"
ISBN 978-0-9559269-0-7

"Blinded by the Bling??" is a short factual book about the destruction of a Site of Special Scientific Interest in order to build a housing development and golf course in the North East of Scotland. This book takes the reader from the first approaches of the developer through the early stages of the planning process up to the point at which a Public Local Inquiry was about to start in the summer of 2008.

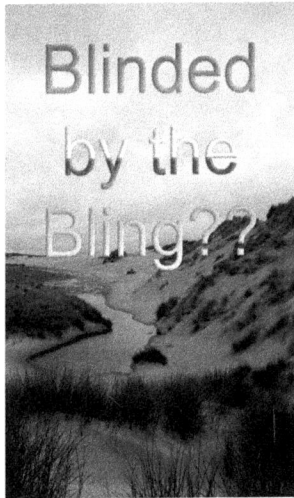

"It's Only  Sand"
ISBN 978-0-9559269-1-4

"It's Only Sand" is a fictional novel set in an imaginary coun-
try not far from here where a foreign multi billionaire developer arrives with the intention of building 'the best resort in the
world' assuming that his 'usual methods' will work just as well
as anywhere else; but he hasn't bargained on the locals and
their determined attitude. So who wins out in the end? Is it the
international developer or the easy going, relaxed locals?

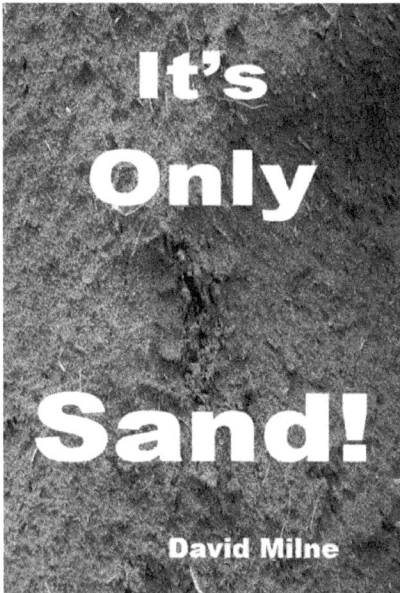